The Mediterranean Diet Cookbook

A Fantastic Collection of Delicious Recipes on the Mediterranean Diet for Beginners. Start Eating Healthy by Rebalancing the Nutrients Essential to your Body's Well-Being.

Angelica Esposito

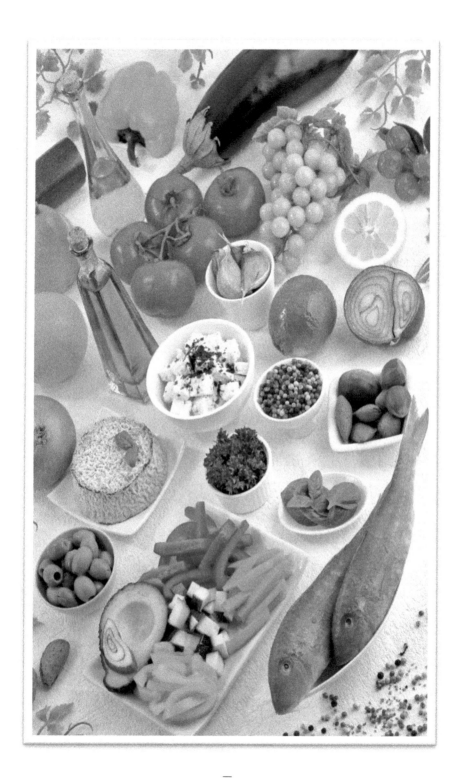

TABLE OF CONTENTS

INTRODUCTION

It is a known fact that eating a balanced diet is important. It's one of the biggest factors in maintaining a healthy lifestyle. But sometimes,, it can be hard to identify what that "well-balanced diet" even looks like. Many people think they are eating healthily while they are just overindulging in the wrong things or not getting enough nutrients from their food. That's dangerous for the body – and can be dangerous for the wallet too!

The Mediterranean diet is a healthy diet that will keep your body healthy while still allowing you to enjoy your favorite foods. The Mediterranean diet emphasizes whole, fresh foods and usually has less than 30% of calories from fat, much lower than average North American diets. One of these food groups is the olive tree fruit and its oil. The Mediterranean diet recommends using olive oil over butter and other oils. Olive oil is rich in mono-unsaturated fatty acids and antioxidants. Because of these benefits, the Mediterranean diet has become very popular in the U.S.

The Mediterranean way of eating isn't just about food; it's also about lifestyle and culture. It stresses physical activity as well as a focus on family, friends, and work-life balance. It encourages people to get outdoors and enjoy the fresh air, and it provides a good foundation for physical and psychological well-being.

There is no concrete Mediterranean diet. The general principles of this diet can be found in the Dietary Guidelines for Americans. These guidelines recommend increasing whole grains, fruits, vegetables, unsaturated fatty acids (found naturally in olives), and monounsaturated fatty acids (found naturally in olive oil) while limiting foods with trans-fat content butter and other oils balance. It also encourages slow, simple cooking. The Mediterranean diet also is high on whole grains, fruits, vegetables, and beans. These foods have been shown to reduce the risk of heart disease and cancer while promoting a healthy brain. It includes nuts and seeds as well as lean meat and fish.

There are many misconceptions about the Mediterranean diet. For example, many people believe eating fish is a healthy part of the diet because it's on the list of foods that make up the Mediterranean diet. However, the Mediterranean diet doesn't include fish as one of its food groups because it can be highly processed. It also contains a lot of salt, too much, and too little is a recipe for heart disease.

In addition to its great health benefits, the Mediterranean diet also has positively affected the economy in Greece and others areas in Europe where it originated. Countries like France have figured out how to make money from olive oil instead of importing it elsewhere. This has helped to stabilize world markets and keep them in this region.

The Mediterranean diet is not a fad. It's a lifestyle that has been around since the days of the ancient Greeks and Romans, and it's one of the reasons they were so healthy. It's easy to see why the Mediterranean diet is a great way to nourish your body and mind.

BREAKFAST

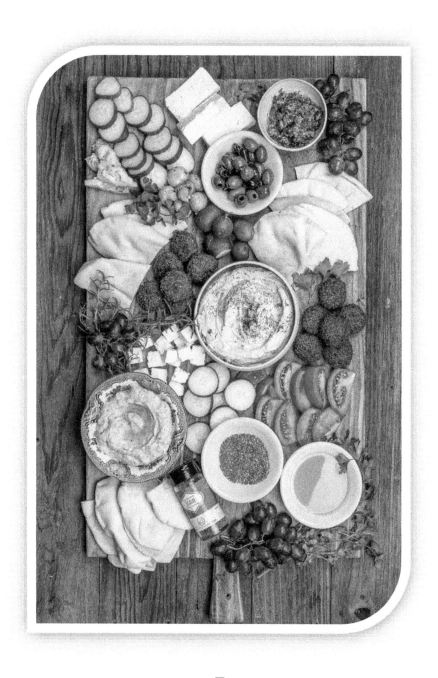

PIZZA WAFFLES

❖ Preparation Time:
❖ Servings: 2

INGREDIENTS

➢ 3 tbsp. Almond Flour
➢ 4 tbsp. Parmesan Cheese
➢ 1 tbsp. Psyllium Husk Powder
➢ 3 oz. Cheddar Cheese
➢ 1 tbsp. Butter
➢ 1 tsp. Baking Powder
➢ 14 slices Pepperoni (optional)
➢ 4 large Eggs
➢ 1 tsp. spices of choice as Seasoning
➢ 1/2 cup Tomato Sauce
➢ Salt and Pepper to Taste

PREPARATION

1. Add all ingredients to a container except for tomato sauce and cheese.
2. Use an immersion blender to blend until the mixture thickens for about 30-45 seconds.
3. Apply heat to your waffle iron and add half of the mixture to the waffle iron.
4. Cook until steam is surfacing off the waffle iron.
5. Once done, move from the iron and repeat with the second half of the mixture. Add tomato sauce and cheese

on the top of each waffle. Then, broil for 3-5 minutes in the oven.

6. Add pepperoni to the top of these if you desire. Once the cheese is melted and starting to crisp on top, remove it from the oven and serve.

NUTRITION

Caloriesn526, Protein 29g, Carbs 5g, Fats 45g

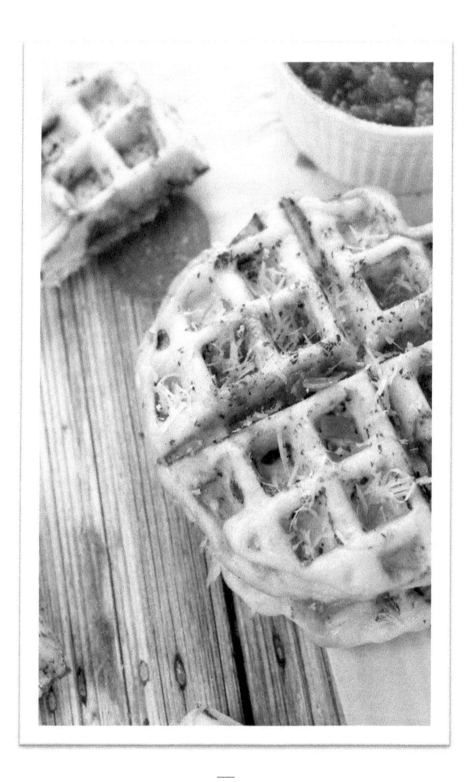

CAULIFLOWER RICE BOWL

❖ Preparation Time: 10 minutes
❖ Servings: 6

INGREDIENTS

➢ 1 cup cauliflower rice
➢ 3 cups broccoli, chopped wild
➢ 1 1/2 tsp curry powder
➢ 1 cup vegetable stock
➢ Pepper to taste
➢ 1/2 tbsp ginger, grated
➢ Salt to taste
➢ 4 tomatoes, chopped
➢ 1/2 tsp red pepper flakes

PREPARATION

1. Spray the interior of the instant pot using cooking spray.
2. Add and stir all ingredients into the instant pot.
3. Close pot with lid and cook on high for 12 minutes.
4. Once done, allow to release pressure naturally for 10 minutes, then release what left using quick release.
5. Remove lid, Stir and serve.

NUTRITION

Calories 44, Carbohydrates 8.2 g, Protein 2.8 g, Fat 0.8 g

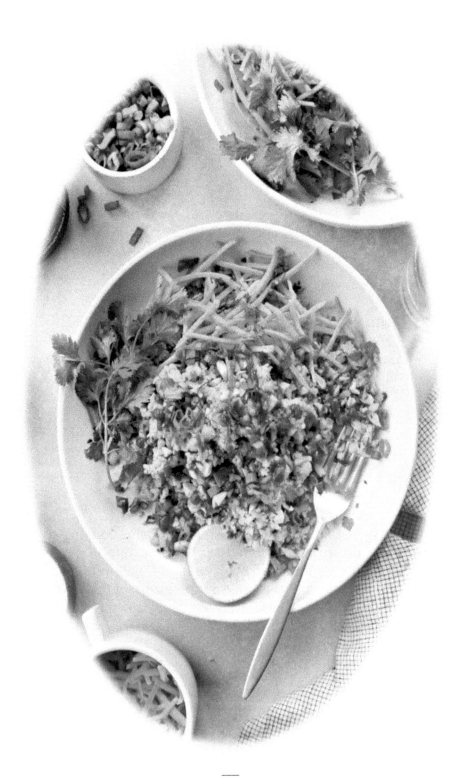

MINI PANCAKE DONUTS

❖ Preparation time:
❖ Servings: 8

INGREDIENTS

➤ 3 OZ. Cream Cheese
➤ 4 tbsp. Almond Flour
➤ 1 tsp. Vanilla Extract
➤ 10 drops Liquid Stevia
➤ 1 tsp. Baking Powder
➤ 1 tbsp. Coconut Flour
➤ 4 tbsp. Erythritol
➤ 3 large Eggs

PREPARATION

1. Place all ingredients inside a container and mix using an immersion blender until it becomes a smooth batter that's slightly thickened.
2. Heat the donut maker and spray with coconut oil. Introduce batter into each well of the donut maker, filling about 90% of the way.
3. Cook for 3 minutes on one side, then flip and cook for an extra 2 minutes.
4. Remove donuts from the donut maker once they are done and set them aside to cool.
5. Repeat the process with the rest of the batter.

NUTRITION

Calories 32, Carbs 0.4g, Protein 4g, Fats 7g

FRITTATAS MINI

❖ Preparation time: 5 minutes
❖ Servings: 12

INGREDIENTS

➤ 1 yellow onion, chopped
➤ A drizzle of olive oil
➤ 1 yellow bell pepper, chopped
➤ 1 red bell pepper, chopped
➤ 2 tablespoons chives, chopped
➤ 1 cup parmesan, grated
➤ Salt and black pepper to the taste
➤ 8 eggs, whisked
➤ 1 zucchini, chopped

PREPARATION

1. Apply medium-high heat to a pan with the oil.
2. Add the onion, the zucchini, and the rest of the ingredients except the eggs and chives and sauté for 5 minutes, stirring often.
3. Divide the mix on the bottom of a muffin pan, pour the eggs mixture on top, sprinkle salt, pepper, and chives, and bake at 350 degrees F for 10 minutes.
4. Serve.

NUTRITION

Calories 95.5g, Protein 4.2g, Carbohydrates 3.2g, Fat 3g, Fiber 0.7g

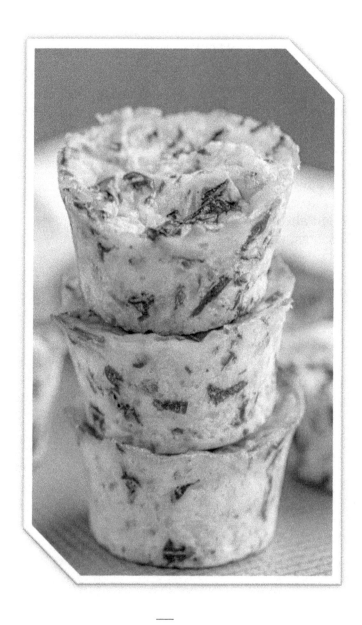

JALAPENO POPPER EGG CUPS

❖ Preparation Time:
❖ Servings: 4

INGREDIENTS

➤ 12 strips Bacon
➤ 8 large Eggs
➤ 4 oz. Cheddar Cheese
➤ 3 oz. Cream Cheese
➤ 4 medium Jalapeno Peppers, de-seeded and chopped
➤ 1/2 tsp. Garlic Powder
➤ 1/2 tsp. Onion Powder
➤ Salt and Pepper to Taste

PREPARATION

1. Measure out all cheese and grate as desired.
2. Chop the jalapenos and them. Keep 1 jalapeno cut into rings as a garnish for the top.
3. Preheat the oven to 375F.
4. Cook the bacon so it's semi crisp. Keep the bacon grease in the pan.
5. Using a hand mixer, mix eggs, cream cheese, chopped and seeded jalapeno peppers, leftover bacon grease, garlic powder, onion powder, and salt and pepper to taste.
6. Grease the wells of the muffin tin, then place par-cooked bacon around the edges.

7. Pour the egg mixture into the muffin tin's wells. Make sure you just go around half to two-thirds of the way up because they are very steep.
8. Place a slice of cheddar cheese on top of the muffin, followed by jalapeno. Cook for 20-25 minutes at 375°F.
9. Once cooked, remove from the oven and allow to let cool for a while.

NUTRITION

Calories 216, Protein 6g, Carbs 0.9g, Fats 13g

COBBLER

- ❖ Preparation Time: 10 minutes
- ❖ Servings: 4

INGREDIENTS
- ➤ 2 lbs. apples, cut into chunks
- ➤ 1/4 tsp nutmeg
- ➤ 1/2 cup dry buckwheat
- ➤ Pinch of ground ginger
- ➤ 1/2 tsp cinnamon
- ➤ 1/2 cup dates, chopped
- ➤ 1/2 cups water

PREPARATION

1. Spray the interior of an instant pot using cooking spray.
2. Add and stir all ingredients into the instant pot.
3. Cover and set timer for 12 minutes.
4. Once done, release pressure using quick release.
5. Remove lid, stir and serve.

NUTRITION

Calories 195, Protein 3.3 g, Carbohydrates 48.3 g, Fat 0.9 g

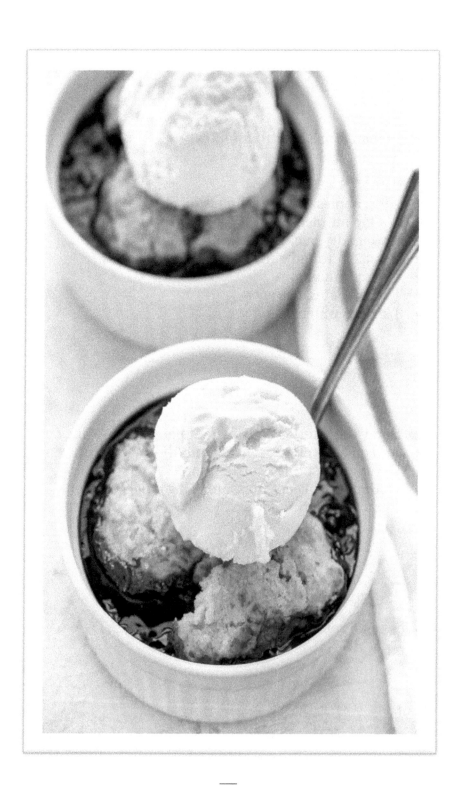

PANCAKE SANDWICH

❖ Preparation Time:
❖ Servings: 1

INGREDIENTS

➢ 0.75 oz. Pork Rinds
➢ 2 oz. Hot Sausage
➢ 1/4 tsp. Vanilla Extract
➢ 1 tbsp. Heavy Cream
➢ 1 tbsp. Almond Flour
➢ 1 large Egg, beaten
➢ The Filling
➢ 1 slice Cheddar Cheese
➢ 2 tbsp. Maple Syrup

PREPARATION

1. In a food processor, pulverize pork rinds until a powder forms.
2. On the burner, heat a pan to medium-high heat.
3. Cook the sausage in a ring mold until it reaches a medium-well temperature. Set aside in foil to rest until cooked.
4. Mix pork rinds with all bun ingredients while the sausage is cooking.
5. Fill the pan 3/4 of the way with bun batter using an egg ring mold.

6. Remove the ring mold until the bottom of the bun has browned and flipped to the other side. Cook until this side is browned as well.
7. Using the other half of the batter, repeat the process.
8. In the same pan, lightly scramble an egg in the ring mold. Cook until the mixture is fully solidified.
9. Assemble with 1 bun on the bottom, 1 slice of cheese, hot egg, sausage, and the last bun on top. Then, serve!

NUTRITION

Calories 657, Protein 40g, Carbs 7g, Fats 57g

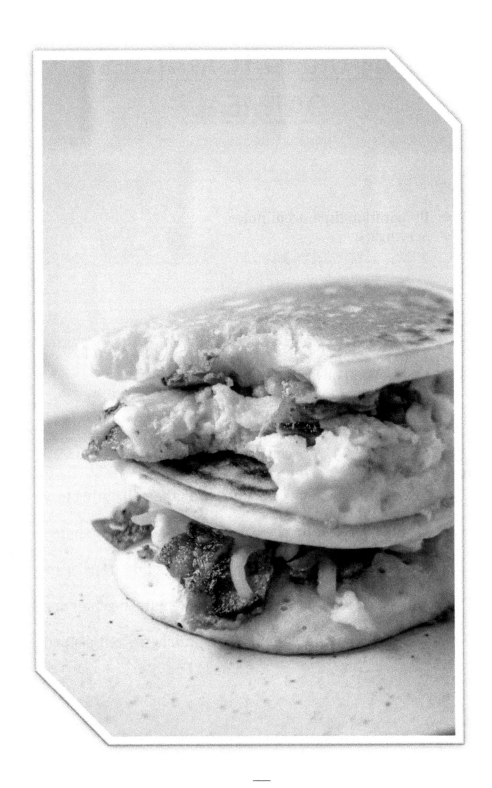

SUN-DRIED TOMATOES OATMEAL

❖ Preparation time: 10 minutes
❖ Servings: 4

INGREDIENTS

➢ 1 cup steel-cut oats
➢ 1 tablespoon olive oil
➢ 1 cup almond milk
➢ A pinch of red pepper flakes
➢ ¼ cup sun-dried tomatoes, chopped
➢ 3 cups water

PREPARATION

1. In a pan, add and mix the water with the milk, bring to a boil over medium heat.
2. Meanwhile, heat up the pan with the oil over medium-high heat.
3. Add the oats, cook for about 2 minutes and transfer to the pan with the milk.
4. Add tomatoes and simmer over medium heat for 23 minutes.
5. Divide the mixture into dishes, sprinkle the red pepper flakes on top, and serve.

NUTRITION

Calories 170, Protein 1.5, Carbohydrates 3.8, Fat 17.8, Fiber 1.5

LUNCH

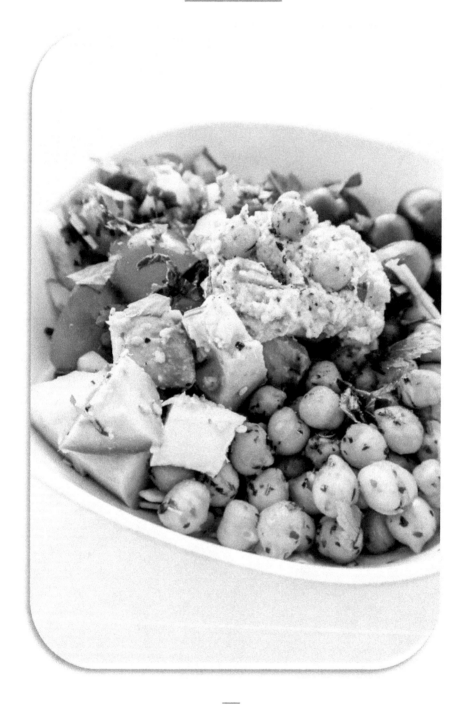

MIXED GREEN SPRING SALAD

- ❖ Preparation Time:
- ❖ Servings: 1

INGREDIENTS

- ➢ 2 OZ. Mixed Greens
- ➢ 2 slices Bacon
- ➢ 3 tbsp. Pine Nuts, roasted
- ➢ Salt and Pepper to taste
- ➢ 2 tbsp. Shaved Parmesan
- ➢ 2 tbsp. 5 Minute Raspberry Vinaigrette

PREPARATION

1. Cook bacon until very crisp
2. Measure out your greens and set them in a container that can be shaken.
3. Crush bacon, then add the other ingredients to the greens. Agitation the container with a lid on to distribute the dressing and contents evenly.

NUTRITION

Calories 478, Fat 33g, Carbs 3g, Protein 11g.

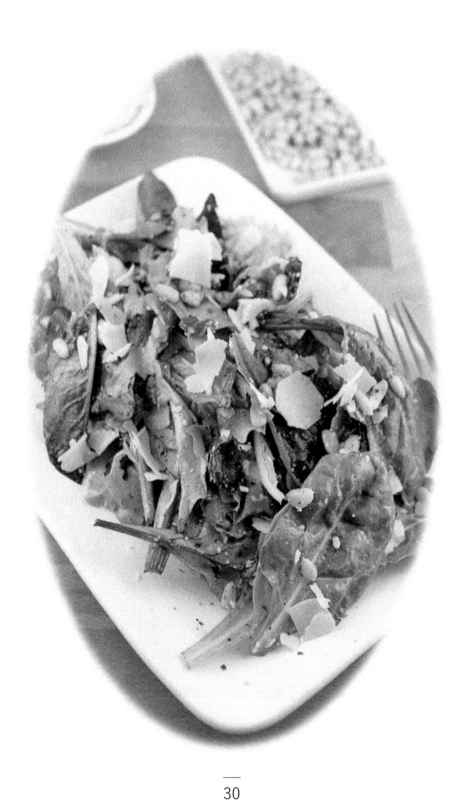

MINTY LAMB STEW

- ❖ Preparation time: 10 minutes
- ❖ Servings: 4

<u>INGREDIENTS</u>

- ➢ 2 pounds lamb shoulder
- ➢ 15 ounces canned chickpeas
- ➢ 28 ounces canned crushed tomatoes
- ➢ ½ cup mint, chopped
- ➢ 1 tablespoon grated ginger
- ➢ 3 tablespoons olive oil
- ➢ 1 carrot, chopped
- ➢ 1 cup apricots, dried and halved
- ➢ 2 cups orange juice
- ➢ 1 celery rib, chopped
- ➢ 6 tablespoons Greek yogurt
- ➢ 1 tablespoon garlic, minced
- ➢ ½ cup mint, chopped
- ➢ 1 yellow onion, chopped
- ➢ Salt to the taste
- ➢ black pepper to the taste

<u>PREPARATION</u>

1. Place your pot over medium-high heat, add and heat up 2 tablespoons of oil.
2. Add the meat and brown for 5 minutes. Add the carrot, onion, celery, garlic, and ginger, stir and sauté for 5 minutes more.

3. Then, add what is left of the ingredients without the yogurt, bring to a boil, and cook over medium heat for 1 hour and 30 minutes.
4. Split the stew into dishes, top each portion with the yogurt and serve.

NUTRITION

calories 355, protein 15.4, carbs 22.6, fat 14.3, fiber 6.7

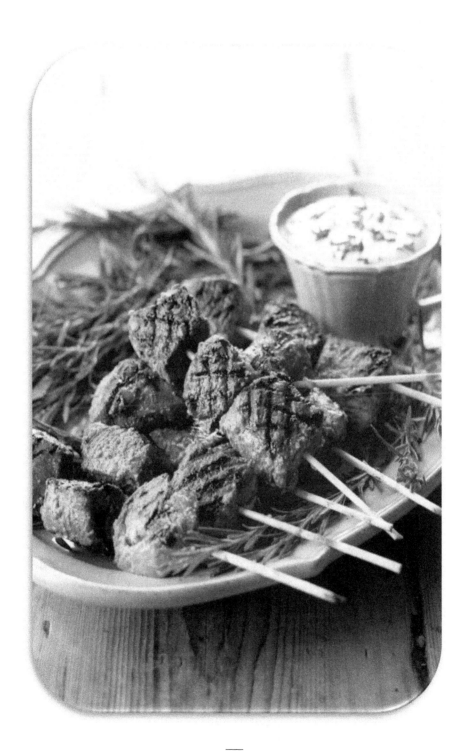

EGG DROP SOUP

- ❖ Preparation Time:
- ❖ Servings: 1

INGREDIENTS

- ➤ 1 1/2 cups Chicken Broth
- ➤ 2 large Eggs
- ➤ 1 tbsp. butter
- ➤ 1/2 cube Chicken bouillon
- ➤ 1 tsp. Chili Garlic Paste

PREPARATION

1. Put a pan on the cooktop and turn it up to a medium-high.
2. Add in the chicken broth, bouillon cube, and butter.
3. Bring the broth to a boil mixing the whole thing together. Then, add the chili garlic paste and stir again. Turn it off.
4. Beat the eggs in a separate container and pour them into the steaming broth.
5. Stir the mixture properly and set aside for a moment to cook.
6. It was once done! Serve up after cooking for 5minutes.

NUTRITION

Calories 279, Protein 12g, Carbs 5g, Fats 23g

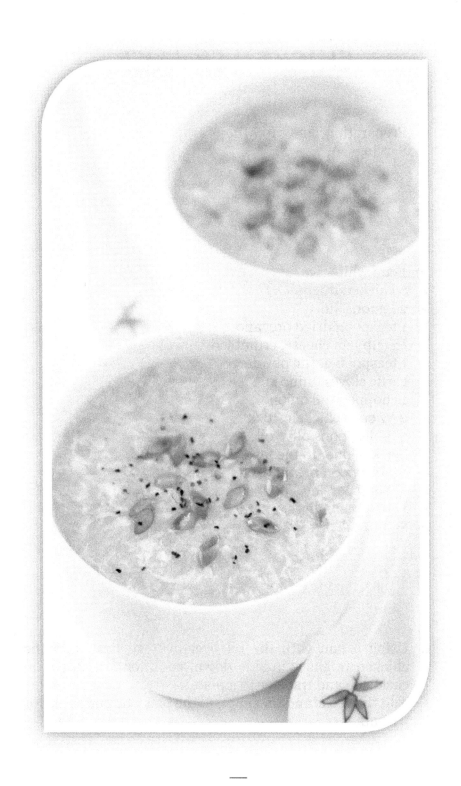

CHICKEN SKILLET

❖ Preparation Time: 10 Minutes
❖ Servings: 6

INGREDIENTS

➢ 1 cup white rice
➢ 6 chicken thighs
➢ 2 lemons Juice
➢ 1 teaspoon dried oregano
➢ ½ cup feta cheese, crumbled
➢ 1 teaspoon garlic powder
➢ garlic cloves, minced
➢ 1 chopped red onion
➢ 2 ½ cups chicken stock
➢ 2 tablespoons olive oil
➢ black pepper to the taste
➢ 1 tablespoon oregano, chopped
➢ 1/3 cup parsley, chopped
➢ 1 cup green olives, pitted
➢ Salt to the taste

PREPARATION

1. Using a pan with the oil over average heat, add the chicken thighs skin side down, cook for 4 minutes on each side and transfer to a plate.
2. Add the garlic and the onion to the pan, stir and sauté for 5 minutes.

3. Then, add the rice, salt, pepper, the stock, oregano, and lemon juice, stir, cook for 1-2 more minutes and take off the heat.
4. Add the chicken to the pan, put the pan into the oven, and bake at 375 degrees F for 25 minutes. Add the cheese, olives, and parsley,
5. Split the whole mix between dishes and serve.

NUTRITION

calories 435, protein 25.6 carbs 27.8, fiber 13.6, fat 18.5

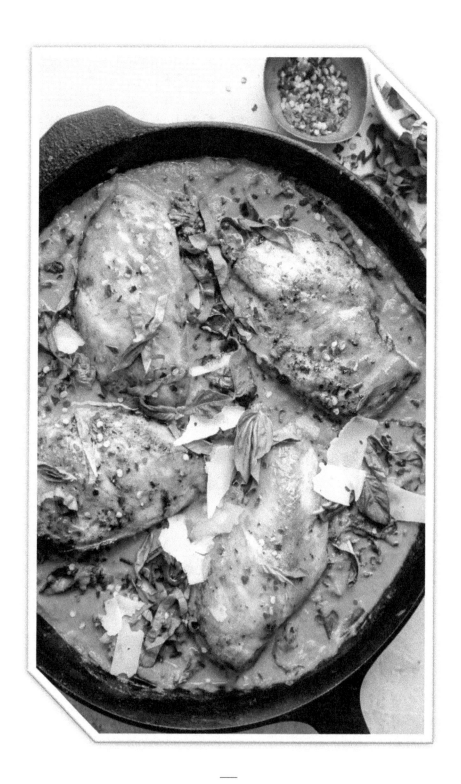

SAUSAGE AND PEPPER SOUP

- ❖ Preparation Time:
- ❖ Servings: 6

INGREDIENTS

- ➢ 32 oz. Pork Sausage
- ➢ 1 can Tomatoes w/ Jalapenos
- ➢ 1 tbsp. Olive Oil
- ➢ 3/4 tsp. Kosher Salt
- ➢ 1 medium Green Bell Pepper
- ➢ 1 tbsp. Cumin
- ➢ 1 tsp. Italian Seasoning
- ➢ 1 tsp. Onion Powder
- ➢ 1 tbsp. Chili powder
- ➢ 4 cups Beef Stock
- ➢ 1 tsp. Garlic Powder
- ➢ 10 oz. Raw Spinach

PREPARATION

1. Apply medium heat to olive oil in a large pot. Once the oil is hot, add in the sausage and fry on one side; mix it to allow it to cook slightly.
2. Meanwhile, add the sliced peppers and stir all together properly. Season with salt and pepper.
3. Add and stir the tomatoes and jalapenos from the can.
4. Then, on top of that, add the spinach and cover the pot.
5. Cook until spinach is wilted, about 6-7 minutes.

6. Cook for around 6-7 minutes, or until the spinach has wilted.
7. Open the lid from the pan and let simmer for 15 minutes longer.

NUTRITION

Calories: 526, Protein: 28g Carbs: 8g, Fats: 43g

CHICKPEAS AND MILLET STEW

❖ Preparation time: 10 minutes
❖ Servings: 4

INGREDIENTS

➢ 14 ounces canned chickpeas
➢ 1 cup millet
➢ 14 ounces canned chopped tomatoes
➢ 2 cups water
➢ 1 yellow onion, chopped
➢ 3 garlic cloves, minced
➢ A pinch of salt and
➢ 2 tablespoons harissa paste
➢ 1 bunch chopped cilantro
➢ 1 eggplant, cubed
➢ 2 tablespoons olive oil
➢ 1 pinch black pepper

PREPARATION

1. Put the water in a pan, bring to a simmer over medium heat, add the millet, simmer for 25 minutes, take off the heat, fluff with a fork and leave aside for now.
2. Heat up another pan with half of the oil over medium heat, add the eggplant, salt, and pepper, stir, cook for 10 minutes and transfer to a container.

41

3. Add what is left of the oil to the pan, heat up over medium heat again, add the onion and sauté for 10 minutes.
4. Add the garlic, more salt, and pepper, the harissa, chickpeas, tomatoes and return the eggplant, stir and cook over low heat for 15 minutes more.
5. Transfer the millet into dishes, toss, divide the mix, sprinkle the cilantro on top, and serve.

NUTRITION

calories 671, protein 27.1 carbs 87.5, fat 15.6, fiber 27.5.

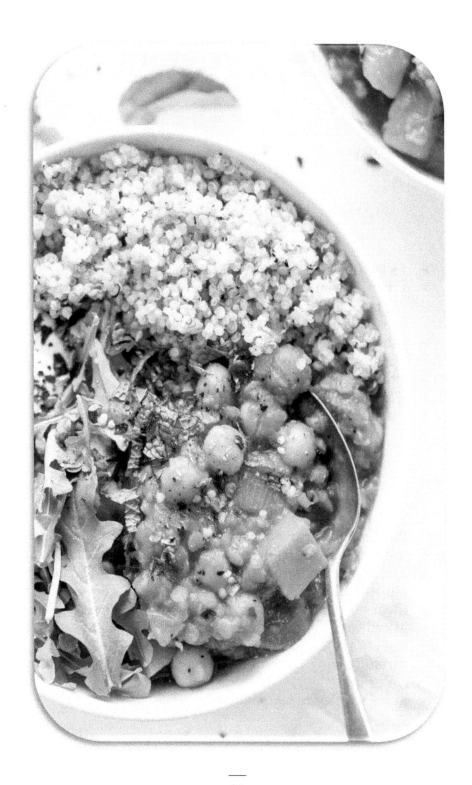

JALAPENO POPPER MUG CAKE

❖ Preparation Time: 25 minutes
❖ Servings: 1

INGREDIENTS

➢ 1 slice Bacon
➢ 1 tbsp. Cream Cheese
➢ 1/4 tsp. Salt
➢ 1 tbsp. butter
➢ 1 tbsp. Golden Flaxseed Meal
➢ 1/2 medium Jalapeno Pepper
➢ 2 tbsp. Almond Flour
➢ 1/2 tsp. Baking Powder
➢ 1 large Egg

PREPARATION

1. Put a pan over average heat and cook the sliced bacon until crisp. Then, pull from the pan and set it aside.
2. Mix in a container all the ingredient with bacon fat(optional)
3. Clear off excess batter on the sides of the container.
4. Microwave the butter for 75 seconds on high at a power level of 10.
5. carefully bang the cup onto the plate to bring the mug cake out.
6. Serve with extra jalapeno.

NUTRITION

Calories: 429, Protein: 15g Carbs: 2g, Fats: 38g.

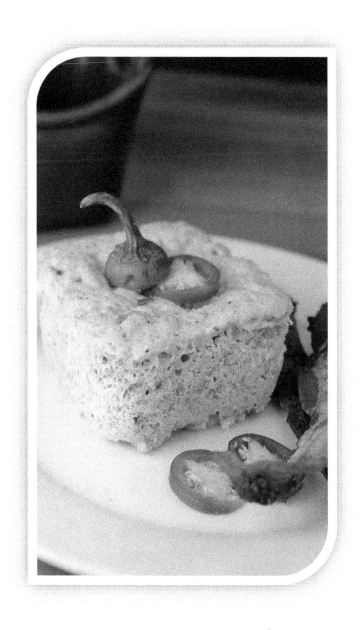

BRUSSELS SPROUTS SALAD WITH CRUNCHY CHICKPEAS

❖ Preparation Time:10 Minutes
❖ Servings:4

INGREDIENTS

➢ 9-ounce shredded Brussels sprouts
➢ 1 cup roasted chickpea
➢ 1 medium avocado
➢ 1/2 cup Tahini Sauce
➢ 4 cups chopped kale

PREPARATION

1. Split Brussels sprouts and kale mix among 4 serving containers with lid.
2. Distribute 2 tablespoons tahini sauce each into the 4 containers
3. Cover the lid refrigerate for up to 4 days.
4. After 4 days of refrigeration, drizzle with 1 portion of tahini sauce and toss well to coat.
5. Top with 1/4 cup roasted chickpeas and 1/4 avocado and serve.

NUTRITION

carbohydrates 30.6g 337 calories; protein 11.9g;

DINNER

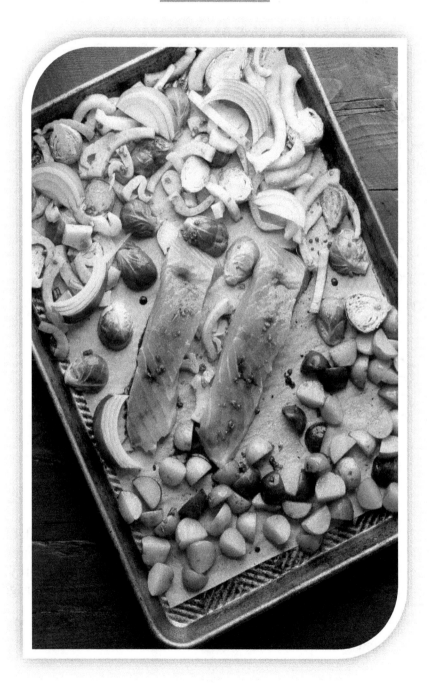

SALMON WITH TARRAGON DILL CREAM SAUCE

❖ Preparation Time: 10 mins
❖ Servings: 8

INGREDIENTS
Salmon Filets
  ➢ 1 1/2 lb. Salmon Filet
  ➢ Pepper to Taste
  ➢ 3/4-1 tsp. Dried Dill Weed
  ➢ 3/4-1 tsp. Dried Tarragon
  ➢ 1 tbsp. Duck Fat
  ➢ Salt to Taste

Cream Sauce:
  ➢ 2 tbsp. Butter
  ➢ Pepper to Taste
  ➢ 1/2 tsp. Dried Dill Weed
  ➢ 1/2 tsp. Dried Tarragon
  ➢ Salt to Taste
  ➢ 1/4 cup Heavy Cream

PREPARATION

1. In a container, slice the salmon in half to create filets. Season fish with tarragon, dill weed, and salt and pepper. Turn around and season skin with salt and pepper only.
2. Heat 1 tbsp. Duck fat in a pan of your choice over average heat. Once hot, add salmon skin side down.
3. Salmon should be cooked for 4-6 minutes. Reduce the heat to low and flip the salmon once the skin is crisp.

4. Cook the salmon until it reaches the desired level of doneness. In most cases, 7-15 minutes on low heat is appropriate.
5. Remove the salmon from the pan and place it on a plate. Allow the butter and spices to be brown in the pan. When the butter has browned, add the cream and stir all together.
6. Serve with broccoli or asparagus, and make sure to eat a lot of it.
7. Garnish with a small number of red pepper flakes.

NUTRITION

Calories: 469, Fats: 40g, Carbs: 5g, Protein: 25g.

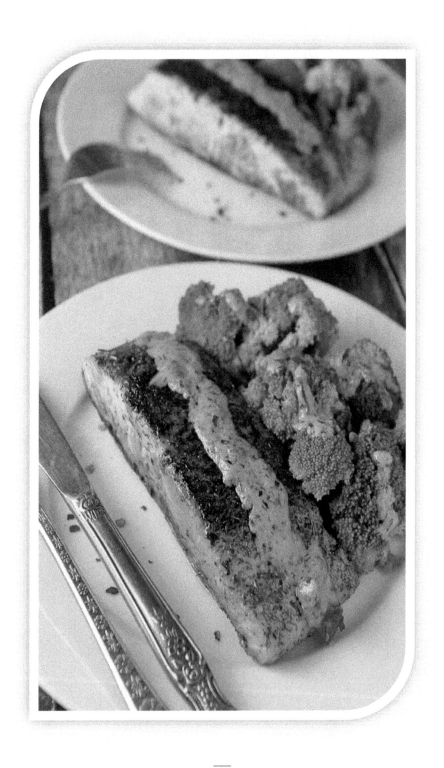

RIBEYE STEAK

- ❖ preparation Time: 15 Minutes
- ❖ Servings: 2

INGREDIENTS

- ➢ 16 oz. Ribeye Steak
- ➢ 1 tbsp. Butter
- ➢ Pepper to Taste
- ➢ 1 tbsp. Duck Fat
- ➢ Salt to Taste
- ➢ 1/2 tsp. Thyme, chopped

PREPARATION

1. First, more the cast iron skillet into the oven by Preheating it at 400F.
2. Rub with a light coating of duck fat and also apply a coating layer of salt and pepper on all sides, including the edges.
3. Once done with the pre-heating, take away the cast iron skillet and place it on the stovetop over medium heat. Add duck fat, and put your steak into the pan, and scorch for 1 1/2 to 2 minutes.
4. Flip the steak and put it into the oven immediately for 4-6 minutes.
5. Take the steak out of the oven and place it on the stovetop over low heat.

6. Add the butter to the pan and base the steak with the butter. Scoop the batter with a spoon, spreading it over the steak for 2-4 minutes
7. , cover, and give it time to rest for 5 minutes. Serve with your preferred veggies.

NUTRITION

Calories: 750, Protein: 38g, Carbs: 0g, Fats: 66g.

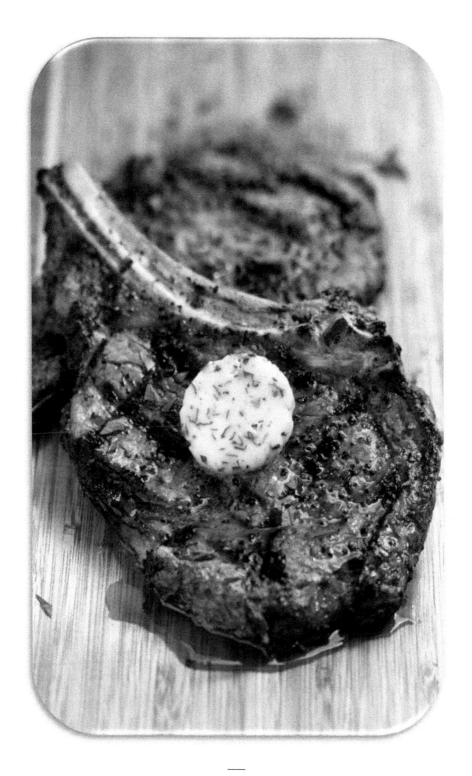

CREAMY BUTTER SHRIMP

* ❖ Preparation Time:
* ❖ Servings: 3

INGREDIENTS

- ➤ 1/2 oz. Parmigiano Reggiano, grated
- ➤ 1 tbsp. Water
- ➤ 1/2 tsp. Baking Powder
- ➤ 1 large Egg
- ➤ medium Shrimp
- ➤ 3 tbsp. Coconut Oil
- ➤ 1/4 tsp. Curry Powder
- ➤ 2 tbsp. Almond Flour

Creamy Butter Sauce:
- ➤ 2 small Thai Chilies, sliced
- ➤ 2 tbsp. Unsalted Butter
- ➤ 1 clove Garlic, finely chopped
- ➤ 1/2 small Onion, diced

Garnish:
- ➤ 1/8 tsp. Sesame Seeds
- ➤ Salt to Taste
- ➤ 1/2 cup Heavy Cream
- ➤ /3 oz. Mature Cheddar
- ➤ 12 tbsp. Curry Leaves
- ➤ Pepper to Taste

PREPARATION

1. In a container, add 0.5 oz. Grated Parmigiano Reggiano, almond flour, baking powder, and curry powder (optional) and them all together.
2. Moderately cut the surface of the shrimps and strip. Add into the mixture, add in 1 egg and 1 tbsp. Water and mix until smooth.
3. Preheat a pan on medium heat. Add in 3 tbsp. Coconut oil. Once the oil is hot, coat the shrimps with the batter and pan-fry the shrimps. Repeat two to three times.
4. Once the shrimps turn golden brown and remove them from the pan, put them on a cooling rack. Pan-fry extra batter if any left.
5. In the pan over medium-low heat. Add in unsalted butter, and the moment the butter has melted enough, add in the chopped onion.
6. Cook until the onion turns translucent, and then add in finely chopped garlic, sliced Thai chilies, and 2 tbsp. Curry leaves. Stir-fry everything until fragrant.
7. Add in the battered shrimp and coat well with the sauce.
8. Serve with cauliflower fried rice and sesame seeds on top.

NUTRITION

Calories: 570, Protein: 14g, Carbs: 3g, Fats: 52g

ROASTED TURKEY LEGS

❖ Preparation Time: 15 Minutes
❖ Servings: 4

INGREDIENTS

➤ 2 medium Turkey Legs
➤ 1/2 tsp. Dried Thyme
➤ 1/2 tsp. Pepper
➤ 1/2 tsp. Onion Powder
➤ 1 tsp. Worcestershire
➤ 2 tsp. Salt
➤ 1/2 tsp. Ancho Chili Powder
➤ 1 tsp. Liquid Smoke
➤ 1/4 tsp. Cayenne Pepper
➤ 1/2 tsp. Garlic Powder

PREPARATION

1. Add and mix the dry ingredients into a small container. Then, add in and mix them together with the wet ingredients into a rub.
2. Dry the turkey legs with paper towels completely. Then, apply on the turkey leg a layer of seasoning.
3. Pure in 2 tbsp. Of fat to medium-high heat in a skillet. Add turkey legs into the pan and scorch on each side for 1-2 minutes.
4. Place in the oven at 350F until cooked through or for 50-60 minutes.
5. Remove turkey from the oven and cool for a few minutes.

6. Serve with your favorite side dish.

NUTRITION

Calories: 382, Protein: 44g Carbs: 0.8g, Fats: 25g.

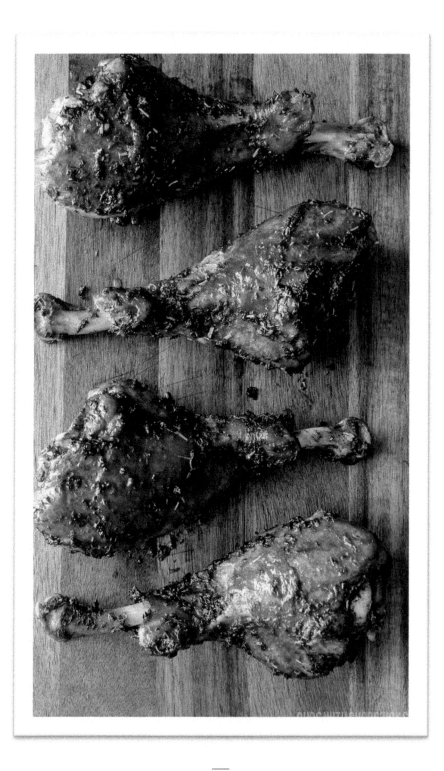

STUFFED MEATBALLS

* ❖ Preparation Time: 25 Minutes
* ❖ Servings: 4

INGREDIENTS

- ➢ 1 1/2 lb. Ground Beef
- ➢ 1/2 tsp. Italian Seasoning
- ➢ 3 tbsp. Tomato Paste
- ➢ 1/2 cup sliced Olives,
- ➢ 1 tsp. Worcestershire Sauce
- ➢ 3 tbsp. Flaxseed Meal
- ➢ 1/2 cup Mozzarella Cheese
- ➢ 1 tsp. Oregano
- ➢ 2 tsp. Minced Garlic
- ➢ Salt to Taste
- ➢ Pepper to Taste
- ➢ 2 large Eggs
- ➢ 1/2 tsp. Onion powder

PREPARATION

1. In a large mixing container, add your ground beef, oregano, Italian seasoning, and garlic and onion powder. Mix all together using your hands
2. Add in the eggs, tomato paste, flaxseed, Worcestershire, and mix again.
3. Finally, cut your olives into small pieces and combine them with the shredded mozzarella cheese in your beef. All should be mixed together.

4. Apply heat to the oven up to 400 degrees Fahrenheit and begin forming the meatballs. In all, you'll have about 20 meatballs. Place on a foil-lined cookie sheet.
5. Bake the meatballs in the oven for 16-20 minutes or until baked to your liking.
6. Serve with a plain spinach salad on the side and a drizzle of the cookie sheet fat.

NUTRITION

Calories 594, Protein38g, Carbs 8g, Fat s48g

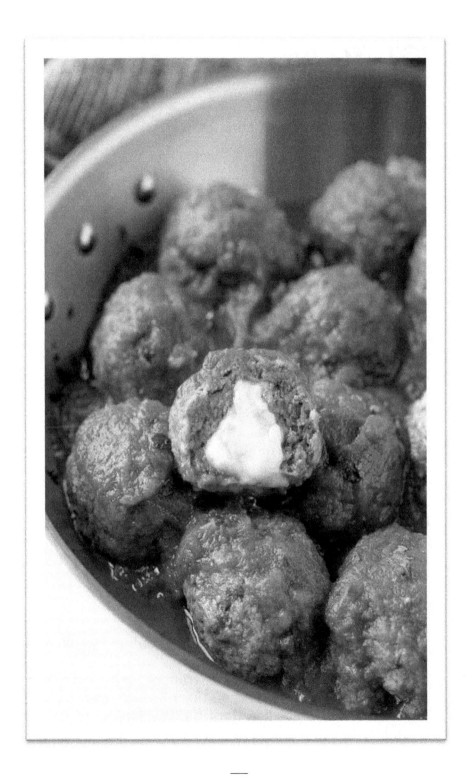

POTATO AND CHICKEN STEW

- ❖ Preparation Time: 10 minutes
- ❖ Servings: 4

INGREDIENTS

- ➢ 1-pound golden potatoes, diced
- ➢ 1 ½ pounds chicken legs
- ➢ 1 cup red onions, chopped
- ➢ 1/2 teaspoon cumin seeds
- ➢ 2 carrots, peeled and sliced
- ➢ Sea salt to taste
- ➢ 2 cups roasted vegetable broth
- ➢ 1 thyme sprig
- ➢ 1/2 teaspoon ginger, peeled and minced
- ➢ 1/2-pound green beans, trimmed
- ➢ 2 tablespoons olive oil
- ➢ 2 bay leaves
- ➢ 1 rosemary sprig
- ➢ 3 cloves garlic, peeled
- ➢ freshly ground black pepper to taste

PREPARATION

1. apply medium-high heat to 1 tablespoon of the olive oil in a Dutch oven.
2. Cook the cumin seeds until fragrant or for 30 seconds.
3. Then, heat what is left of the olive oil and fry the vegetables and chicken until the vegetables are tender and the chicken is no longer pink.

4. Add in the garlic, ginger, and spices, and cook further for an additional minute or so.
5. Discharge in the broth and stir to combine. Next, turn the heat to a simmer for 30 minutes or until heated through.
6. Shred the chicken with two forks and add it back to the Dutch oven. Stir in the green beans and let it simmer until crisp-tender for 4 minutes.

NUTRITION

Calories: 405; Protein: 38.8g; Carbs: 27.9g; Fat: 14.9g

PROTEIN-PACKED CHICKEN BEAN RICE

❖ Preparation Time: 10 Minutes
❖ Servings: 6

INGREDIENTS

➢ 1 lb. chicken breasts, cut into chunks
➢ 4 cups chicken broth
➢ Salt to taste
➢ 2 cups brown rice
➢ 1 tbsp olive oil
➢ 1 tbsp Italian seasoning
➢ 14 oz can cannellini beans
➢ Pepper to taste
➢ 1 tbsp garlic, chopped
➢ 1 small onion, chopped

PREPARATION

1. Pure oil into the inner pot of an instant pot and set on sauté mode.
2. Add garlic and onion and sauté for 3 minutes.
3. Include in what is left of the ingredients and stir well. Seal pot and set timer for 12 minutes.
4. Once done, release pressure using quick release. Remove lid, stir well and serve.

NUTRITION

Calories 494, Protein 34.2 g, Carbohydrates 61.4 g, Fat 11.3 g.

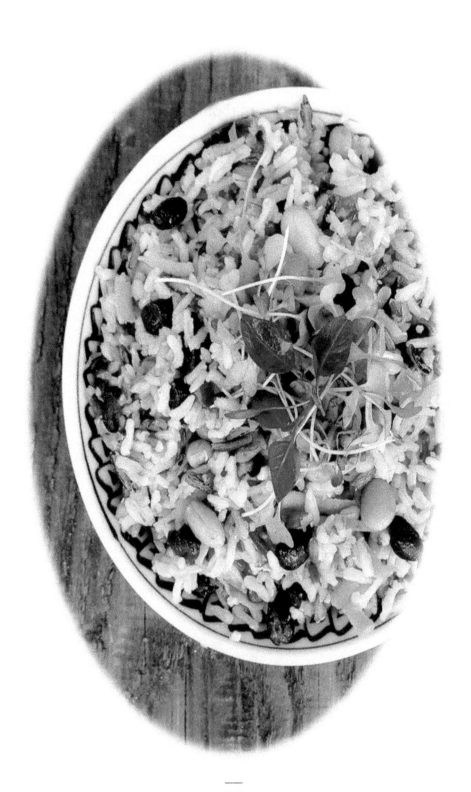

BASIL FISH CURRY

- ❖ Preparation Time: 10 Minutes
- ❖ Servings: 4

INGREDIENTS

- ➤ 10 oz tilapia fillets, chopped
- ➤ 1/2 tsp turmeric
- ➤ 1 tsp ground cumin
- ➤ 1 1/2 tsp chili powder
- ➤ 1 tsp ground coriander
- ➤ 1/2 cup fresh basil, chopped
- ➤ 1 tsp fresh lemon juice
- ➤ Salt to taste
- ➤ 3 tbsp olive oil
- ➤ 1 chili pepper, chopped
- ➤ 1/2 cup grape tomatoes, chopped
- ➤ 2 cups of coconut milk
- ➤ 1 tsp garlic, minced
- ➤ 1 small onion, chopped

PREPARATION

1. Pure in oil into the pot of instant pot and set on sauté mode.
2. Add onion, salt, garlic, and all spices, and cook for 2-4 minutes. Add coconut milk and stir well.
3. Add fish, grape, tomatoes chili pepper, and stir properly. Seal pot with lid and boil on high for about 4 minutes.

4. Once done, release pressure using quick release. Remove lid. Stir in basil and serve.

NUTRITION

Calories 444; Protein 16.7 g; Carbohydrates 10.5 g; Fat 40.2 g; Sugar 5.5 g.

SNACKS

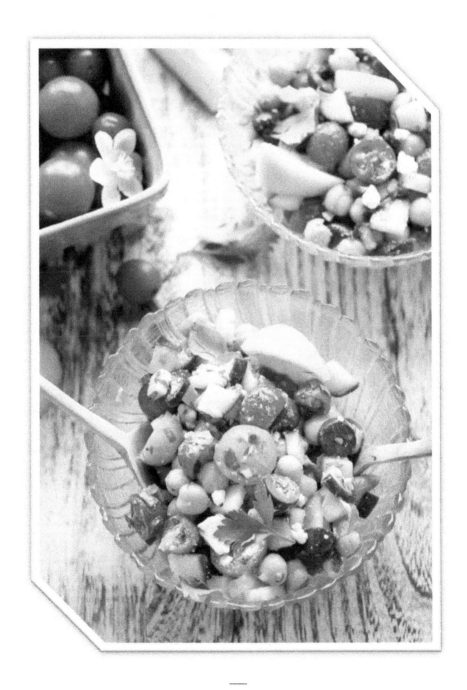

COCONUT ORANGE CREAMSICLE BOMBS

- ❖ Preparation Time: 5 Minutes
- ❖ Servings: 10

INGREDIENTS

- ➤ 1/2 cup Coconut Oil
- ➤ 1 tsp. Orange Vanilla Mio
- ➤ drops Liquid Stevia
- ➤ 4 oz. Cream Cheese
- ➤ 1/2 cup Heavy Whipping Cream

PREPARATION

1. Microwave all ingredients leaving out liquid stevia and Orange Vanilla for about a minute
2. Blend microwaved ingredients Using an immersion blender
3. Stir in liquid stevia and Orange Vanilla Mio into the mix.
4. Spread into a tray and refrigerate in a freezer for 2-3 hours.
5. Once frozen, remove from tray and stock in the freezer.

NUTRITION

Calories 176, Protein 0.8g, Carbs 0.7g, Fats 20g.

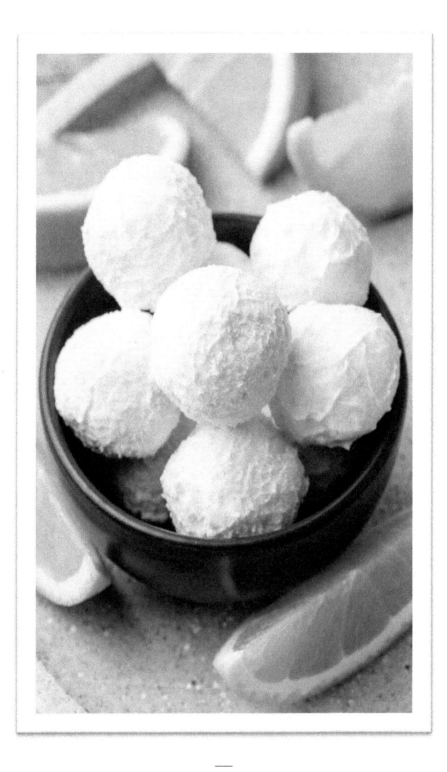

LIME CUCUMBER MIX

❖ Preparation Time: 10 Minutes
❖ Servings: 8

INGREDIENTS

➢ 4 cucumbers, chopped
➢ ½ cup green bell pepper, chopped
➢ 1 garlic clove, minced
➢ 1 chili pepper, chopped
➢ black pepper to taste
➢ 1 yellow onion, chopped
➢ 1 tablespoon olive oil
➢ 1 teaspoon parsley, chopped
➢ 2 tablespoons lime juice
➢ 1 tablespoon dill, chopped
➢ Salt to taste

PREPARATION

1. In a large container, add and mix the cucumber with the bell peppers and
2. Add the other ingredients with the mix, toss and serve.

NUTRITION

calories 123, protein 2, carbs 5.6, fat 4.3, fiber 2.3

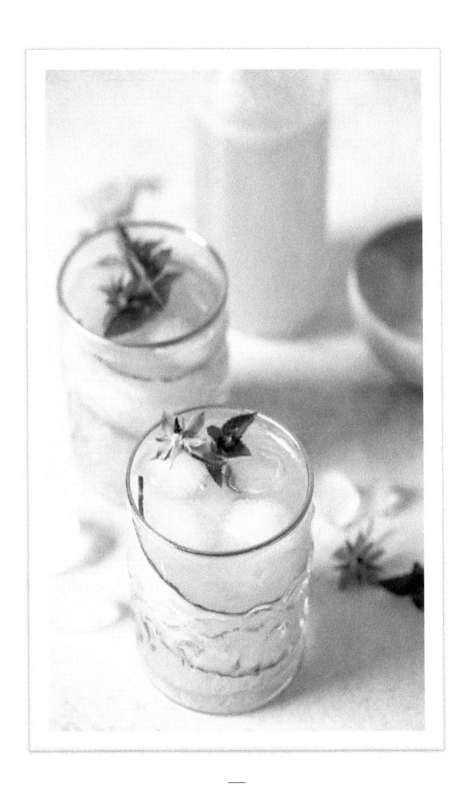

CREAMY POTATO SPREAD

- ❖ Preparation Time: 10 Minutes
- ❖ Servings: 6

INGREDIENTS

- ➤ 1 lb. sweet potatoes, chopped
- ➤ 1 cup tomato puree
- ➤ Pepper to taste
- ➤ 3/4 tbsp fresh chives, chopped
- ➤ Salt to taste
- ➤ 1 tbsp garlic, minced
- ➤ 1/2 tsp paprika

PREPARATION

1. Pure all ingredients apart from chives into the inner pot of instant pot and stir to combine as possible.
2. Seal pot with lid and heat on high for 15 minutes.
3. Next, release pressure naturally for 10 minutes, then releases remaining using quick release.
4. Remove lid. Transfer the mixture into the food processor and pulse until smooth.
5. Garnish with chives and serve.

NUTRITION

Calories 108; Protein 2 g; Carbohydrates 25.4 g; Fat 0.3 g; Sugar 2.4 g.

TORTILLA CHIPS

- ❖ Preparation Time: 10 Minutes
- ❖ Servings: 6

INGREDIENTS

- ➢ Tortilla Chips:
- ➢ 12 oz Flaxseed Tortillas
- ➢ Salt to Taste
- ➢ 3 tbsp. Absorbed Oil
- ➢ Pepper to Taste
- ➢ Optional Toppings:
- ➢ Full-Fat Sour Cream
- ➢ Fresh Salsa
- ➢ Diced Jalapeno
- ➢ Shredded Cheese

PREPARATION

1. Heat ready your deep fryer
2. Cut each tortilla into 6 chip-sized slices and lay the pieces in the basket of a deep fryer.
3. Fry 4-6 pieces tortilla in the preheated deep fryer for about 1-2 minutes. Then, flip and fry for another 1-2 minutes on the other side.
4. Once done, move from the fryer and cool on a paper towel. Season to your desired taste with salt and pepper.
5. Serve with your preferred toppings

NUTRITION

Calorie 147, Protein 0.9g, Carbs 0.04g, Fats 1g

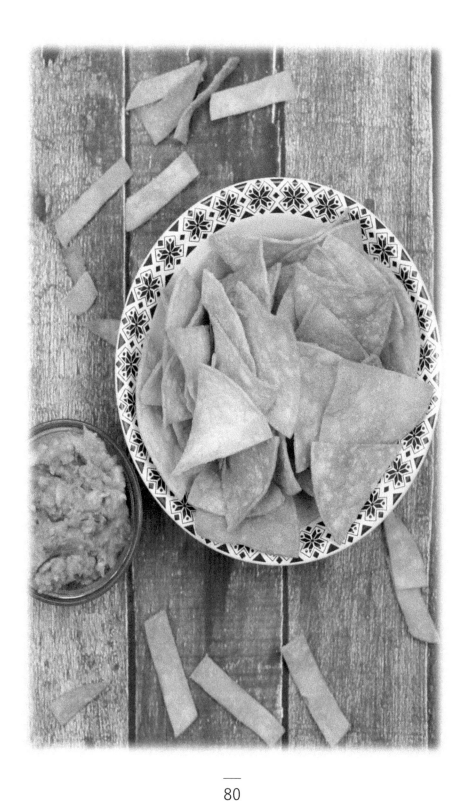

CORNDOG MUFFINS

- ❖ Preparation Time: 10 Minutes
- ❖ Servings: 6 To 10

INGREDIENTS

- ➢ 10 Let's Smokies
- ➢ 1/2 cup Flaxseed Meal
- ➢ 1/3 cup Sour Cream
- ➢ 1 tbsp. Psyllium Husk Powder
- ➢ 1/2 cup Blanched Almond Flour
- ➢ 1/4 cup butter, melted
- ➢ 1/4 cup Coconut Milk
- ➢ 1/4 tsp. Baking Powder
- ➢ 3 tbsp. Swerve Sweetener
- ➢ 1 large Egg
- ➢ 1/4 tsp. Salt

PREPARATION

1. Preheat oven to 375F.
2. Add and mix all of the dry ingredients properly in a container.
3. Add egg, sour cream, and butter, and then mix well. Once mixed, add the coconut milk and continue to mix.
4. Divide the batter up between 20 well-greased mini-muffin slots, then cut the Lit'l Smokies in half and stick them in the middle.
5. Bake for 12 minutes and then broil for 1-2 minutes until the tops are lightly browned.

6. Once done, give time to cool on a wire rack.

NUTRITION

Calories 79, Protein 4g, Carbs 0.7g, Fats 8g,

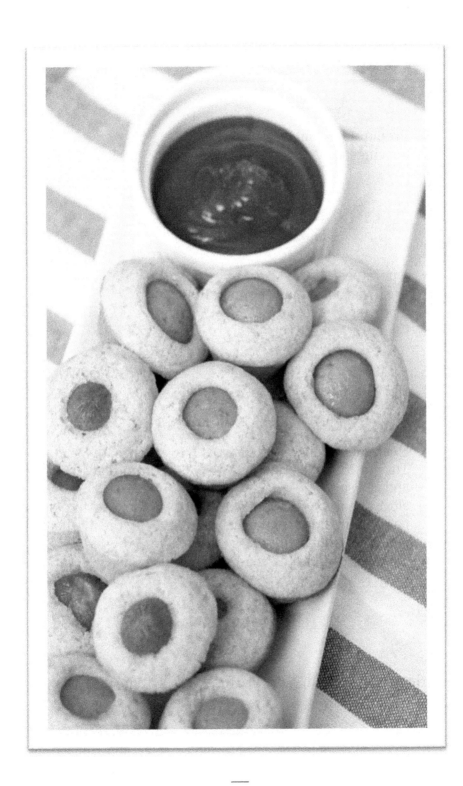

HOMEMADE POTATO CHIPS

- ❖ Preparation Time: 25 minutes
- ❖ Servings: 4

INGREDIENTS

- ➢ 2 potatoes, sliced
- ➢ freshly ground black pepper, to taste
- ➢ 2 tablespoons olive oil
- ➢ Coarse sea salt to taste

PREPARATION

1. Heat your oven to 395 degrees F to get it ready.
2. Toss to coat the potatoes with oil, ground black pepper, and sea salt.
3. Next, position the potatoes in a single coating on a parchment-lined baking sheet. Bake in the preheated oven for about 15 minutes until golden brown.
4. Taste and adjust the seasonings. Enjoy

NUTRITION

Calories: 202; Protein: 3.8g; Carbs: 32.2g; Fat: 6.9g

CABBAGE AND MUSHROOMS MIX

❖ Preparation Time: 10 Minutes
❖ Servings: 2

INGREDIENTS

➢ ½ pound white mushrooms, sliced
➢ 2 tablespoons olive oil
➢ 4 spring onions, chopped
➢ 1 tablespoon balsamic vinegar
➢ 1 yellow onion, sliced
➢ 1 green cabbage head, shredded
➢ Salt to taste
➢ black pepper to taste

PREPARATION

1. Apply medium heat to a pan with the oil.
2. Add spring onions and yellow onion to the heated pan and cook for 5 minutes.
3. Stir in the rest of the ingredients, and cook the whole mix for 10 minutes,
4. After cooking, divide between dishes and serve.

NUTRITION

calories 199, protein 2.2, carbs 5.6, fat 4.5, fiber 2.4.

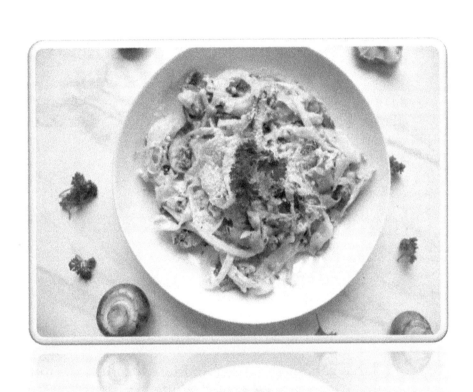

BUCKEYE COOKIES

❖ Preparation Time: 10 minutes
❖ Serves: 4

INGREDIENTS

➢ 2 1/2 Cups Honeyville Almond Flour
➢ 1 Tbsp. Vanilla Extract
➢ 1/2 tsp. Salt
➢ 2-3 Choco perfection Bars
➢ 1/4 Cup Coconut Oil
➢ 3 Tbsp. Maple Syrup
➢ 1/4 Cup Now Erythritol
➢ 1 1/2 tsp. Baking Powder
➢ 1/2 Cup Peanut Butter

PREPARATION

1. In a large container, add in and mix together 1/4 Cup Coconut Oil, 1/2 Cup Peanut Butter, 1 Tbsp. Vanilla Extract and3 Tbsp. Maple Syrup with a hand mixer.
2. In a separate container, mix up 2 1/2 Cups Honeyville Almond Flour, 1/4 Cup now Erythritol, 1 1/2 tsp. Baking Powder, and 1/2 tsp. Salt. Transfer to wet mix using a sifter. Mix all until it forms a crumbled dough.
3. Use your hands to mix the dough into a ball. Cover the ball in plastic wrap and freeze for 30 minutes.
4. Before getting your dough out, cut up 2 Choco perfection bars into small chunks. You want to fit 1-2 pieces into each cookie.

5. Preheat your oven to 350F. Then, rip off small chunks of dough at a time. Press the chocolate into the dough.
6. Seal the dough with your hands until the chocolate cannot be seen.
7. Press the dough into a rounded shape to achieve consistency. Lay all cookies down on a non-stick baking liner about 1 inch distance from each other. Bake for 15-18 minutes.

NUTRITION

Calories 148, Protein 4g, Carbs 5g, Fats 16g

DESSERTS

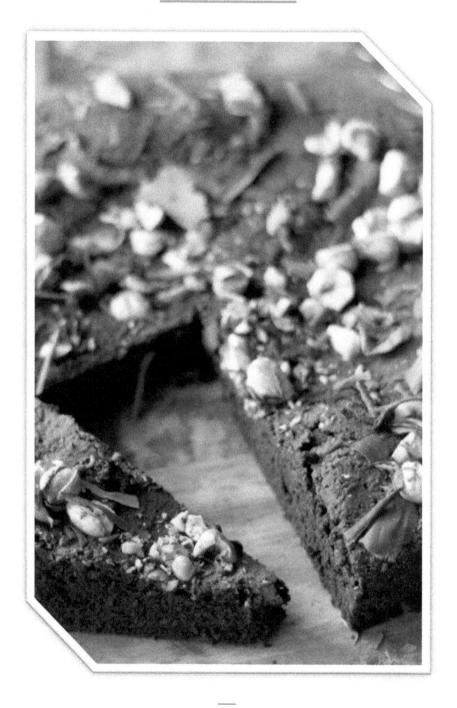

BROWN BUTTER PECAN ICE CREAM

❖ Preparation Time: 10 minutes
❖ Servings: 1 quart

INGREDIENTS

➢ 1 1/2 cups Unsweetened Coconut Milk
➢ 1/4 cup Heavy Cream
➢ 1 cup Butter
➢ 1/4 cup Pecans, crushed
➢ 25 drops Liquid Stevia
➢ 1/4 tsp. Xanthan Gum

PREPARATION

1. In a pan over low heat, stir to melt the butter until it melted and starts to turn a deep amber color.
2. Crush the pecans in a plastic bag and add along with stevia and heavy cream once the butter is brown. Stir together properly.
3. In a container, combine the coconut milk, butter mixture, and xanthan gum. Then combine everything with a whisk.
4. Fill your ice cream machine halfway with the mixture and process according to the manufacturer's instructions.
5. Serve and enjoy!

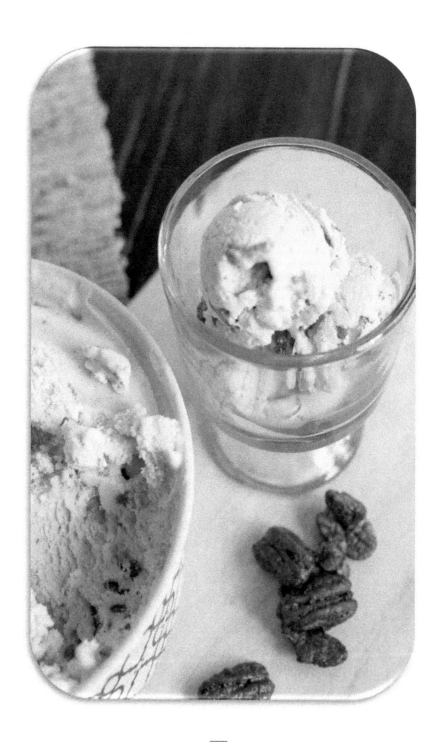

CHOCOLATE SMOOCH FUDGE

❖ Preparation Time: 5 minutes
❖ Servings: 16

INGREDIENTS

➢ 12-ounce vegan semisweet chocolate chips
➢ 2 tablespoons cranberry juice
➢ 1/2 cup sweetened dried cranberries
➢ 2 tablespoons brandy
➢ 1 cup shredded sweetened coconut
➢ 1 cup chopped walnuts

PREPARATION

➢ Fill an 8-inch square baking pan halfway with waxed paper foil, allowing the ends to hang over the pan's edge. Set aside.
➢ In an average pan, gradually melt the chocolate chips over low heat. Stir in the walnuts, coconut, and cranberries. Stir in the brandy, and pulse until smooth.
➢ Scrape the mixture into the organized pan. Smooch evenly and refrigerate for at least 2 hours.
➢ Once cooled, move the fudge from the pan, and transfer it to a board for cutting.
➢ Take and throw away the waxed paper. Cut the fudge into 2-inch pieces and serve.

NUTRITION

Calories 69.9, Protein 0.4g, Carbohydrates 13g, Fat 1.8g, Fibber 0.3g

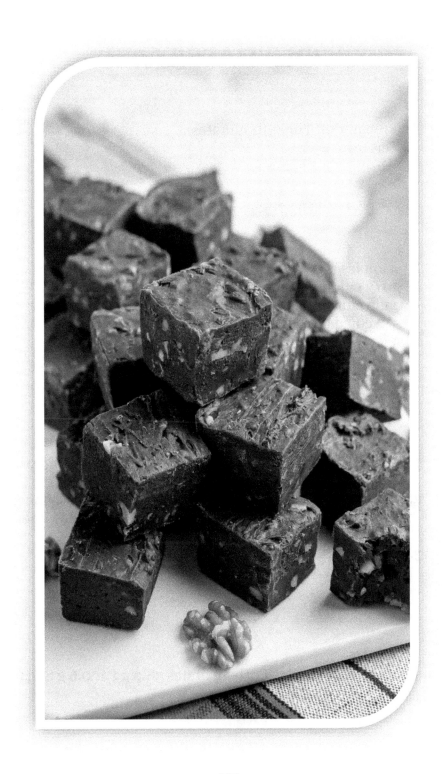

APPLE DATES MIX

- ❖ Preparation Time: 10 minutes
- ❖ Servings: 4

INGREDIENTS

- ➤ 4 apples
- ➤ 1 1/2 cups apple juice
- ➤ 1 tsp cinnamon
- ➤ 1/2 cup dates, pitted
- ➤ 1 tsp vanilla

PREPARATION

1. Add all ingredients into the instant pot inner pot and stir properly.
2. Seal the pot and cook on high for 15 minutes. Once done, allow to release pressure naturally for 10 minutes, then release the residual using quick release.
3. Remove lid. Stir and serve.

NUTRITION

Calories 226 Protein 1.3 g Carbohydrates 58.6 g Fat 0.6 g Sugar 46.4 g

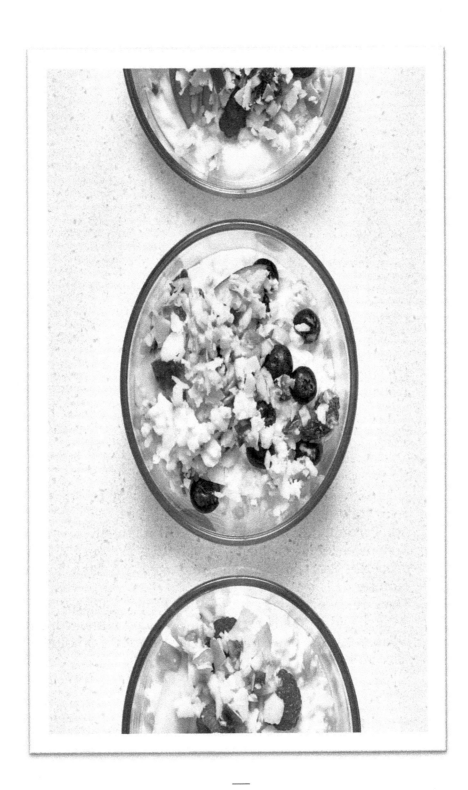

SWEET COCONUT RASPBERRIES

- ❖ Preparation Time: 10 minutes
- ❖ Serve: 12

INGREDIENTS

- ➢ 1/2 cup dried raspberries
- ➢ 1/2 cup shredded coconut
- ➢ 3 tbsp swerve
- ➢ 1/2 cup coconut butter
- ➢ 1/2 cup coconut oil

PREPARATION

1. Set instant pot on sauté mode.
2. Add coconut butter into the pot and let it melt.
3. Add in coconut, raspberries, oil, and swerve and stir properly. Seal pot with lid and cook on high for 2 minutes.
4. Then, release pressure by means of quick release. Take away the lid. Spread berry mixture on a parchment-lined baking tray and place in the refrigerator for 3-4 hours.
5. Slice and serve.

NUTRITION

Calories 101 Protein 0.3 Carbohydrates 6.2 g Fat 10.6 g Sugar 5.1 g

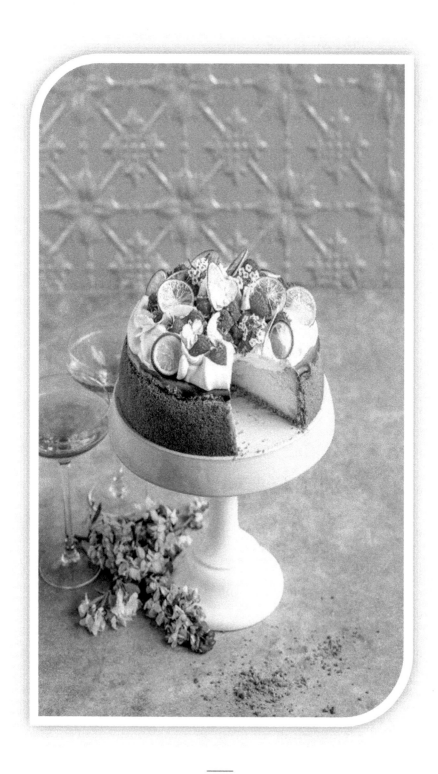

RAISINS CINNAMON PEACHES

- ❖ Preparation Time: 10 minutes
- ❖ Servings: 4

INGREDIENTS

- ➢ 4 cored peaches, cut into chunks
- ➢ 1 cup of water
- ➢ 1 tsp vanilla
- ➢ 1/2 cup raisins
- ➢ 1 tsp cinnamon

PREPARATION

1. Add all the listed ingredients into the internal pot of instant pot and stir properly.
2. Seal with lid and cook on high for 15 minutes.
3. After cooking, give time to release pressure naturally for 10 minutes, then release what is left using quick release.
4. Remove the lid. Stir together and serve.

NUTRITION

Calories 118, Protein 2 g, Carbohydrates 29 g, Fat 0.5 g, Sugar 24.9 g.

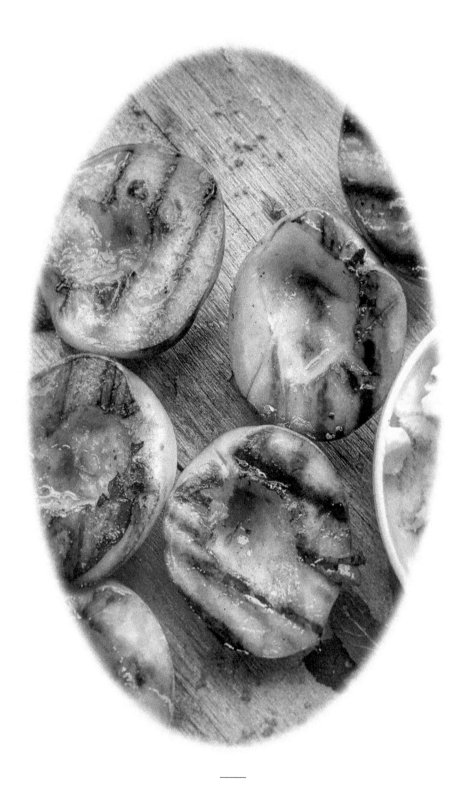

VEGAN WHITE CHOCOLATE

❖ Preparation Time: 5 minutes
❖ Serves: 1

INGREDIENTS

➢ ½ cup food-grade cocoa butter
➢ 2 tablespoons soy milk powder
➢ ½ cup confectioners' sugar
➢ 2 teaspoons pure vanilla extract

PREPARATION

1. Apply oil to a small baking sheet lightly and set it aside.
2. In a medium container, combine the sugar and soy milk powder. Set aside.
3. Melt the cocoa butter in the top of a double boiler over medium heat. Then, stir in the sugar and soy milk mixture and cook, stirring regularly, until the dry ingredients are dissolved, and the mixture is smooth and well blended.
4. Turn off the heat. Mix in the vanilla, stirring until blended.
5. Scrape the batter onto the baking sheet that has been lined with parchment paper and refrigerate to cool completely for about 1 hour.
6. Break into pieces, then transfer to a tightly sealed container and refrigerate until needed.

NUTRITION

Calories 102, Protein 2 g, Carbohydrates 6 g, Fat 8 g, Sugar 4 g.

BANANA-WALNUT CAKE

❖ Preparation Time: 15 Minutes
❖ Servings: 8

INGREDIENTS

➢ 2 ripe bananas
➢ 1⁄2 cup chopped walnuts
➢ 1⁄2 teaspoon ground allspice
➢ 1⁄2 teaspoon ground cinnamon
➢ 2 cups all-purpose flour
➢ 2 teaspoons pure vanilla extract
➢ 3⁄4 cup sugar
➢ 1⁄2 cup vanilla soy milk
➢ 1⁄4 cup canola
➢ 1⁄2 teaspoon salt
➢ 21⁄2 teaspoons baking powder

PREPARATION

1. Preheat the oven to 350°F. Spray an 8-inch square cake pan and set it aside.
2. In a large container, add and mix together the baking powder, flour, allspice, cinnamon, and salt and set aside.
3. In a blender, pour in the oil, bananas, sugar, soy milk, and vanilla and blend until smooth.
4. Add the wet ingredients to the dry ingredients and stir until just moistened. Do not over-mix. Fold in the walnuts.

5. Move the batter into an arranged pan and bake for about 35 to 40 minutes. Give time to cool in the pan for 10 to 15 minutes.
6. Cool a wire rack before cutting.

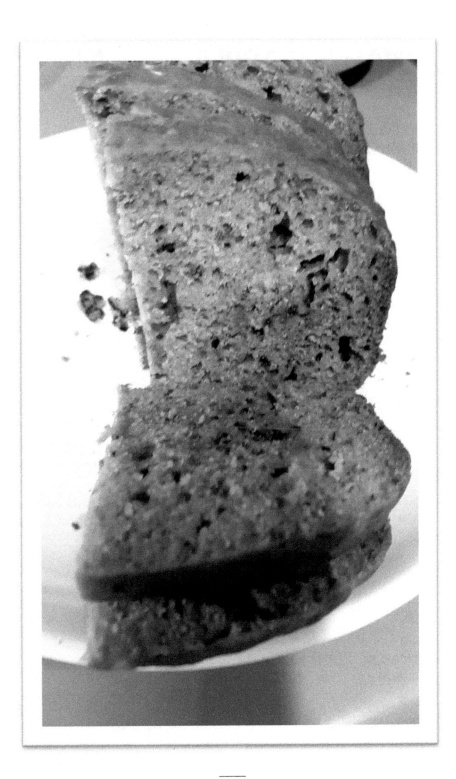

WALNUT APPLE PEAR MIX

- ❖ Preparation Time: 10 minutes
- ❖ Servings: 4

INGREDIENTS

- ➢ 2 cored apples, slice into wedges
- ➢ 1/2 tsp vanilla
- ➢ 1 cup apple juice
- ➢ 2 tbsp walnuts, chopped

PREPARATION

1. Pour all the above ingredients into the inner pot of the instant pot and stir together. Seal pot with lid and cook on high for 10 minutes.
2. Next, allow releasing pressure naturally for 10 minutes, then release remaining using quick release. Remove lid.
3. Serve and enjoy.

NUTRITION

Calories 132, Protein 1.3 g, Carbohydrates 28.3 g, Fat 2.6 g, Sugar 21.9 g

CONCLUSION

The Mediterranean Diet is one of the longest studied diets in history. Adopting this diet has so many benefits an individual can experience. A study revealed that people who assumed the diet were around 30% less likely to die from any cause, mainly because it's a diet rich in healthy fats, whole grains, and produce. People who eat the Mediterranean Diet have low levels of bad (LDL) cholesterol and high levels of good (HDL) cholesterol.

The Mediterranean diet is found to be the best for overall health. It has been shown to reduce heart attack and stroke risk, breast cancer risk, obesity, and overall mortality. The additional benefits of a Mediterranean diet include reduced risk of diabetes, improved control of blood pressure, and possible reductions in risk for dementia and Alzheimer's disease. The diet also comes with health-promoting effects for building bone de

The Mediterranean Diet is a style of eating that originated in Greece and Southern Italy among populations with high levels of physical activity, which includes vegetables, fruit, whole grains, legumes, nuts, and olive oil. The recommendations emphasize foods collected in nature such as fruits and vegetables because they are "nature's food."

In addition, they had lower rates of heart disease and cancer compared to those who eat the Western diet. The diet also may be suitable for people with type 2 diabetes. Feeding yourself and your family healthy meals is a great way to get fit and trim without starving.

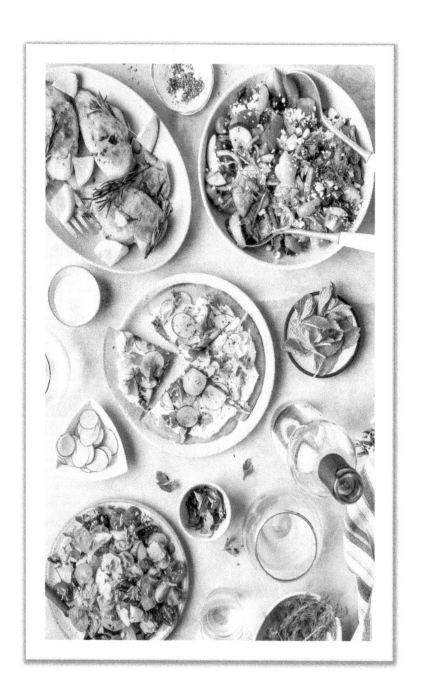

CPSIA information can be obtained
at www.ICGtesting.com
Printed in the USA
BVHW051857130721
611835BV00002B/217